YOUR KNOWLEDGE HAS VALUE

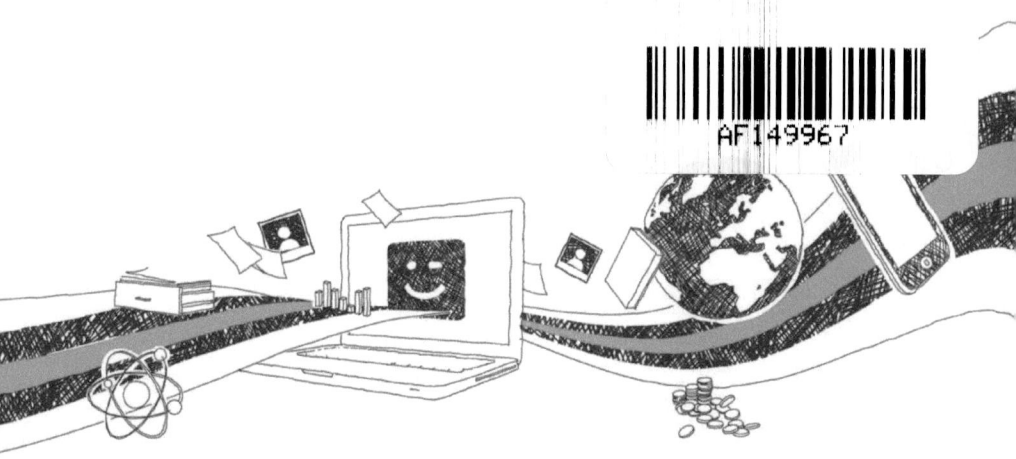

AF149967

- We will publish your bachelor's and
  master's thesis, essays and papers

- Your own eBook and book -
  sold worldwide in all relevant shops

- Earn money with each sale

Upload your text at www.GRIN.com
and publish for free

Bibliographic information published by the German National Library:

The German National Library lists this publication in the National Bibliography; detailed bibliographic data are available on the Internet at http://dnb.dnb.de .

Imprint:

Copyright © 2012 GRIN Verlag, Open Publishing GmbH
Print and binding: Books on Demand GmbH, Norderstedt Germany
ISBN: 9783668299498

This book at GRIN:

http://www.grin.com/en/e-book/340145/a-multiple-objective-decision-analysis-for-terrorism-protection-potassium

Alexandra Barokova, Miroslava Jergusova

A Multiple-Objective Decision Analysis for Terrorism Protection. Potassium Iodide Distribution in Nuclear Incidents

GRIN Publishing

GRIN - Your knowledge has value

Since its foundation in 1998, GRIN has specialized in publishing academic texts by students, college teachers and other academics as e-book and printed book. The website www.grin.com is an ideal platform for presenting term papers, final papers, scientific essays, dissertations and specialist books.

Visit us on the internet:

http://www.grin.com/

http://www.facebook.com/grincom

http://www.twitter.com/grin_com

Institut für Betriebswirtschaftslehre
Innovations- und Technologiemanagement
Kurs im WS 2012

„A Multiple-Objective Decision Analysis for Terrorism Protection: Potassium Iodide Distribution in Nuclear Incidents"

aus der
KFK Health Care Management
OR in Health Care
LV-Nr.: 040736

Table of content

Table register

Illustration register

Abbreviation register

ARS – acute radiation syndrome

KI – potassium iodide

KIPZ – potassium iodide planning zone

MM – mass mailing

ND – no distribution

NRC – National Research Council

RC – reception center

UN – United Nations

VP – voluntary pick up

1. Introduction

This decision analysis was compiled in order to qualitatively and quantitatively assess the different possible potassium iodide (KI) distribution methods for a hypothetical local region. The possibility of the release of radioactive iodine caused by nuclear accidents or terrorist actions makes it crucial to come up with the best distribution methods of KI in order to protect people against thyroid cancer. (Feng and Keller (2006), p. 76-93)

2. Potassium Iodide (KI)

Potassium Iodide, called also „KI" is a salt of stable and not radioactive iodine needed by human body to create thyroid hormones. This kind of chemical is of crucial importance in case of any human exposure to radioactive iodine either by a nuclear accident/incident, the detonation of nuclear weapons or other terrorist actions. It is an effective way to protect population from the risk of thyroid cancer. There are some reasons, why KI instead of other chemicals are used. KI is inexpensive, stable, and readily available with a long-shelf life if stored properly in dry and shady places. In case of any radiological or nuclear event, radioactive iodine may get into the air and be breathed by local population into the lungs or it may also contaminate food and water and get into the human body otherwise. As a result the contamination of human body by radioactive iodine is called „internal contamination". Large amounts of radioiodine can be responsible for the thyroid cell death because of radioiodine´s beta radiation. The radioactive iodine may be absorbed by the gland and cause fatal injuries to it. By taking KI, the stable iodine, in any nuclear accident, the gland absorbs the non-radioactive iodine. The gland becomes full of non-radioactive iodine and will not be able to absorb any more radioactive iodine from the disaster area thus protecting the gland from the risk of thyroid cancer. (National Research Council (2004), p. 19; REMM 2011)

Furthermore it seems very crucial to mention that iodine is a very important part of thyroid hormones and some mental destructions, retardation or cretinism is caused by the deficiency of iodine. Therefore an accurate intake of iodine is a general public goal. The most efficient way how to provide iodine to the public is through the use of iodized salt. As this is not possible in every area of the world, there are other possible methods, such as the ingestion of iodizes oil, iodination of the central water system, addition of iodine to the animal feed, etc.

The probable low dietary iodine intake in Ukraine Chernobyl led to the increased uptake of radioiodine. (National Research Council (2004), p. 16-17)

However KI does not always offer complete protection against thyroid cancer. The success of how well KI blocks radioactive iodine from entering the human gland depends on various circumstances. Firstly, the time span between the contamination of the environment with the radioactive iodine and taking of KI, are essential. The sooner the KI is taken, the better the drug action. As well as this, the time of absorbing the medicine into the blood needs to be taken into account. Finally, the amount of radioactive iodine released into the environment to which population is exposed, substantially influences the success of the KI medicine. The lower the radiation the higher possibility of KI protection. Besides of these facts, KI is able to protect the human body only against thyroid cancer but not against any other types of cancer or illnesses caused by high doses of radiation. (REMM 2011)

The table 1 below describes the connection between the time when the KI is taken and the protection granted by the drug. By administration of 30–200 mg of stable iodine in form of KI short while before or a few minutes after the nuclear accident the uptake of radioiodine into the gland can be blocked for at least 24 hours. The table shows, that even if KI is taken 8 hours after exposure to radioiodine, the normal uptake of 28 % of radioactive iodine, will be reduced by 40 % to an uptake of approx. 16 %. (National Research Council (2004), p. 20-21)

Table 1: Percent Thyroid Protection from radioiodine after a single 130 mg dosage of KI

Time of KI with Respect to Radioiodine Exposure (hours)	Protection Afforded KI Ingestion (% of control)
-96	Very little
-48	~80
-1	~100
0	98
2	80
3	60
8	40
24	16

Source: National Research Council (2004), p. 21

The most vulnerable members of the population as far as thyroid cancer is concerned are unborn children, infants, young children up to 18 years, pregnant and breastfeeding woman and people with low stores of iodine in their gland. Adults older than 40 years have the lowest risk of thyroid injury. Therefore, they should only take KI when instructed by public health officials and when the radioactive contamination is very high. (REMM 2011)

3. Background

The most serious historical chemical releases of the radioiodine were in the nuclear processing plant of Hanford (1940), in the Russian plant Mayak (1940 and 1950), by testing the atmospheric nuclear weapons in 1950 and 1960 as well as by the nuclear reactor casualties in the United Kingdom (Windscale) in 1957 and the former Soviet Union power plant Chornobyl (also known as „Chernobyl"), which will be further described in more detail. The latest nuclear disaster happened in Fukushima (Japan) in March 2011. The Chernobyl disaster is considered by the many experts and the general public to be one of the most serious nuclear catastrophes associated with many harmful consequences. (National Research Council (2004), p. 9; World Nuclear Association 2012)

3.1. Chernobyl nuclear power plant

The Chernobyl nuclear accident in April 1986 in Ukraine was the one and only disaster in the history of commercial nuclear power with radiation-related fatalities. This nuclear disaster was responsible for the largest uncontrollable release of the radioactive iodine into the environment with substantial health, social and economic impact. A number of human errors in combination with the violation of operating rules of the plant, flawed Soviet reactor design, inadequately trained personnel are mentioned to be some of the reasons that caused the disaster. In addition to this the Chernobyl accident is called to be a direct consequence of Cold War and the lack of any safety culture. (World Nuclear Association 2012)

The Chernobyl accident is known as the explosion and destruction of the Chernobyl 4 reactor. During the first three months after the disaster 30 power plant operators and firemen died. One person was killed immediately because of the explosion and another worker died in hospital that day. Acute radiation syndrome (ARS) was diagnosed in more than 237 cases and 28 people out of these died within a few weeks after the accident as a result of ARS. Between

1987 and 2004 another 19 people died. However it has not been proved that these deaths or other mortality or morbidity in the affected area of Belarus, Russia and Ukraine in the next years have occurred because of the Chernobyl disaster. According to the report of the UN Chernobyl Forum Expert Group: „With the exception of thyroid cancer, direct radiation-epidemiological studies performed in Belarus, Russia and Ukraine since 1986 have not revealed any statistically significant increase in either cancer morbidity or mortality induced by radiation". (Bennett, Repacholi, Carr (2006), p.106) On the other hand, the experts admitted that there was a large increase in child thyroid cancer because of the radiation. Fortunately, the early diagnosis made it possible to avert mortality in many cases. (World Nuclear Association 2012)

3.2. Latest nuclear accident in Fukushima

On 11th March 2011 a major earthquake causing approx. 15 meters high tsunami waves was responsible for the shutdown of the cooling and the power supply function of the three Fukushima Daiichi reactors. This resulted in the Fukushima nuclear disaster.

This nuclear accident was not as serious as at the Chernobyl power plant, but it was still responsible for a large number of economic, financial and psychological damage of Fukushima residents and the general public. The extensive release of radionuclides contaminated the air. The population within 20 km radius from the disaster plant needed to be evacuated. Especially residents under 40 years of age must leave the affected area. Local authorities administered stable iodine. The iodine tablets were positioned at evacuation centers. Cleaning up the contaminated water from the reactor became priority. Moreover, there were no radiation casualties (ARS) reported and no harmful health effects were found in 195 345 affected residents living in the vicinity of the Fukushima plant. (World Nuclear Association 2012)

4. Multiple-objective decision analysis for terrorism protection – key insights and main goals

The multiple-objective decision analysis for the distribution of KI in nuclear disasters has been organized by the National Research Council (NRC). A committee of experts, such as thyroid cancer physicians, radioactive safety experts, nuclear power plant safety professionals and experts in emergency management, was managed with the view of working together on a special KI distribution plan for a hypothetical local region. The main aim of the research was to prove how a decision analysis may support health risk assessment and governmental emergency safety plans and help by terrorism protection.

In situations, in which multiple stakeholders with different views, expectations and goals are involved, it seems to be essential to decide on the basis of a multiple-objective decision-modeling. This allows a systematic analysis of a complex situation while taking into account different objectives and opinions. Many of these situations are complicated and associated with serious health and safety outcomes. As well as this, there may be some legal, political, social and resource constraints in the decision process. During the process of multiple-objective decision analysis, the quantification of the performance of each alternative on the targets, is being accomplished. There exist a number of various weighting methods, among which the swing weight method is often used. This weighting method points out the possible performance on an objective, while creating sliders in a Microsoft Excel spreadsheet and moving („swinging") the weight. (Feng and Keller (2006), p. 77-79)

5. Multiple-objective decision analysis process

5.1. Decision Analysis in general

The purpose of creating a decision analysis results from identifying and analyzing possible strategies of a defined problem area with the main goal of choosing the best possible strategy maximizing the defined utilities. These utilities often differ in the various problem areas which are being evaluated. The decision maker may want to maximize the revenue, minimize the cost or fully ignore them and concentrate on maximizing the probability of surviving or achieving a better quality of life. (Schwartz (2003), p. 486f.) No consideration of the overall revenue or costs is used in the case of serious health risks to the public, e.g. in nuclear incidents. (Feng and Keller (2006), p. 80) Besides of these facts it's crucial to point out that decision analysis can be used in all kinds of public health care sector, i.e. primary prevention, secondary prevention and tertiary prevention. Primary prevention can be generally described as the reduction of the risk factors, while the secondary prevention concentrates on the early detection and diagnostics. The tertiary prevention includes the therapy and aftercare. (Schwartz et al. (2003), p. 487)

In this above mentioned decision analysis which is dealing with the distribution of KI in nuclear incidents the multiple-objective decision analysis approach using a decision-under-certainty model was applied, which will be described in the next chapter in more detail.

5.2. Multiple-objective decision analysis in general

Every decision model is an abstraction from reality. In some cases simple models with no real input are sufficient, other help to reflect the reality as good as possible. Multiple-objective decision analysis is very useful when having a set of different objectives together with different stakeholders. They help the decision maker to model, analyze, compare and choose the best decision. The multiple-objective decision analysis has a number of advantages. First of all, the general approach can be used in problem settings that are similar. As well as this, the multiple-objective decision analysis offers flexibility and integrates several stakeholder views in a single model. Moreover it allows to see trade-offs between the stated objectives. (Feng et al. (2008), p. 103)

5.3. Multiple-objective decision analysis for KI distribution

5.3.1. Characteristics of the decision problem

As the KI decision problem is characterized by multiple stakeholders as well as multiple objectives, the multiple-objective decision analysis was used in order to determine the best possible solution. Figure 1 shows the decision analysis approach.

Figure 1: Multiple-Objective Decision Analysis Approach

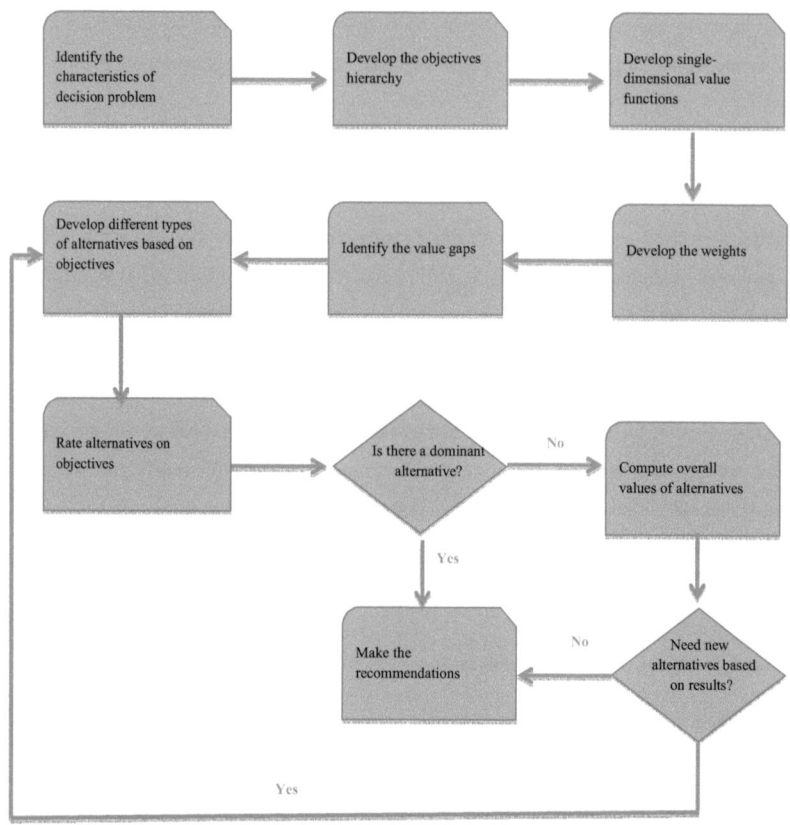

Source: Own representation with reference to Feng and Keller (2006), p. 79

The illustration begins with identifying the characteristics of a decision problem, such as stakeholders or main focus. Then on the one hand it's necessary to develop the objectives hierarchy for the KI decision problem and on the other hand to develop single-attribute value functions, which are helpful when assessing the decision problem. The next step is to set weights for the different objectives developed and to identify the value gaps, which means to identify the difference between the no distribution alternative and the ideal situation. Furthermore alternatives are developed in order to achieve the objectives set. Finally the decision maker will need to rate these alternatives and choose the best one. If there is a clearly dominant strategy, which is not very often the case, it will be recommended. If there is neither the dominant nor the best alternative but instead the need to develop new alternatives, the decision maker will need to go through the process of developing and rating the alternatives again. (Feng and Keller (2006), p. 79-87)

When describing the steps of a multiple-objective decision analysis based on the distribution problem of KI in case of a nuclear incident, it's crucial to identify the characteristics of this decision problem. There are many stakeholders such as government agencies, state and the public involved in this decision problem. Government agencies play a significant role in it as they are the primary institutions that may decide in the end. Besides of this the decision analysis is also characterized by a scientific perspective. It was conducted by experts who were able to provide the whole study with realistic insights. NRC concentrated not only on KI as the best protection from the radioiodine, but also on minimizing harm from other aspects of a nuclear incident. NRC was not of the opinion of involving the cost factor into the decision analysis, as a nuclear incident may have serious health impacts on the inhabitants. These are seen as more important than the cost factor. (Feng and Keller (2006), p. 80)

5.3.2. Objectives Hierarchy

The decision makers need to come up with objectives of the evaluated decision problem. Because the decision problem lies in the health sector, where the safety of the population is of a very high importance, it was not difficult for the stakeholders to agree on them. This was very helpful for understanding the decision problem and evaluating the alternatives chosen. Figure 2 demonstrates the objectives hierarchy.

Figure 2: Multiple-Objective Decision Analysis Approach

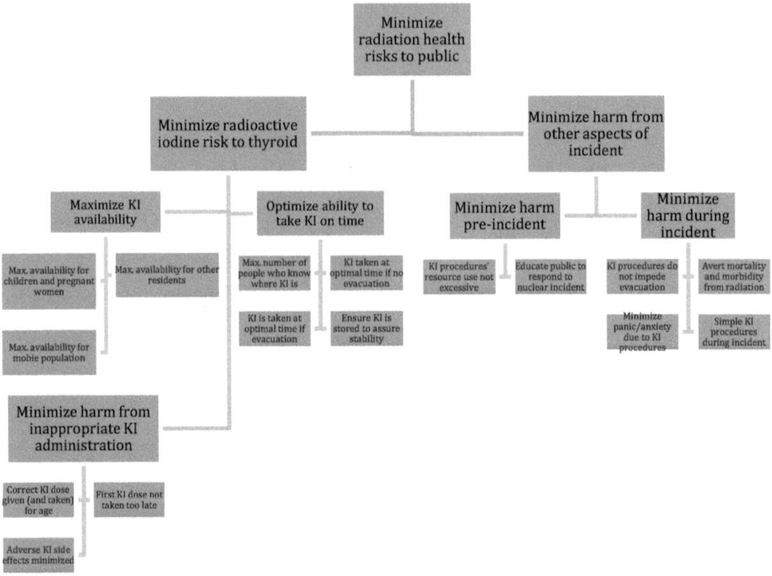

Minimize radiation health risks to public

Minimize radioactive iodine risk to thyroid

Minimize harm from other aspects of incident

Maximize KI availability

Optimize ability to take KI on time

Minimize harm pre-incident

Minimize harm during incident

Max. availability for children and pregnant women

Max. availability for other residents

Max. number of people who know where KI is

KI taken at optimal time if no evacuation

KI procedures' resource use not excessive

Educate public to respond to nuclear incident

KI procedures do not impede evacuation

Avert mortality and morbidity from radiation

Max. availability for mobile population

KI is taken at optimal time if evacuation

Ensure KI is stored to assure stability

Minimize panic/anxiety due to KI procedures

Simple KI procedures during incident

Minimize harm from inappropriate KI administration

Correct KI dose given (and taken) for age

First KI dose not taken too late

Adverse KI side effects minimized

Source: Own representation with reference to Feng and Keller (2006), p. 81

The overall objective is to minimize radiation health risks to the public, followed by two sub-objectives: minimize radioactive iodine risk to thyroid and minimizing harm from other aspects of the incident. These two sub-objectives include five objectives on the third level and another 16 objectives on the lowest level. Although NRC did not include the costs factor into this decision analysis, the objective „KI procedures' resource use not excessive" is partly covering it. Finally it's necessary to point out, that the objectives may vary from one geographical region to the other. The above mentioned structure was developed for a hypothetical region lying near a nuclear power plant. (Feng and Keller (2006), p. 81)

5.3.3. Single-Attribute Value Functions

The multiple-objective decision analysis continues with developing single-attribute value functions. An attribute is considered to be single valued if it consists of one value only. An additive value function is generally speaking suitable for multiple-objective decision analysis, as it is able to combine single-attribute-value functions with weights on the stated objectives. It can be used as follows:

$$v\left(x_1, x_2, \ldots, x_n\right) = \sum_{i=1}^{n} w_i \, v_i \left(x_i\right)$$

Described more in detail v $(x_1, x_2, \ldots, x_n)$ stands for the overall value of an alternative, x_i demonstrates the alternative's performance taking into account the ith objective. Finally w_i represents the weight given to a specific objective and v_i is the single-attribute value function again taking into account the ith objective. Furthermore it is crucial to mention that one objective is fully independent from the other objective. A widely use method in order to develop the single-attribute value function are rating scales as shown in table 2 (Feng and Keller (2006), p. 81-82)

Table 2: Rating scales example

Maximize KI availability			
	x1: Max. availability for children and pregnant women residents	x2: Max. availability for other residents	x3: Max. availability for mobile population
Selected points on 0-10 rating scale vi (xi)			
0	1 dose/person in stockpile	0 doses/person in stockpile	1 dose/child in stockpile
5	50% have extra dose at home now	10% have extra dose at home now	1 dose/person in stockpile
10	85% have extra dose at home	25% have extra dose at home now	25% have extra dose at mobile location now

Source: Own representation with reference to Feng and Keller (2006), p. 82

In the above mentioned illustration, the rating scale reaches the values from 0 to 10, where 0 means the lowest rating option and 10 the exact opposite. If we look at the objective „to maximize availability for other residents", the fact of having 0 doses/person in stockpile will receive the lowest possible rating. 25% of other residents having an extra dose at home now will receive the highest possible rating. This evaluation is again depending from the particular geographical area considered.

5.3.4. Weighs of the objectives

The next step every decision maker will need to go through when doing a multiple-objective decision analysis is to develop weights for the stated objectives. The sum of all developed weights gives a total of 100%. In other words, every decision maker needs to clarify which objectives are most important in the decision problem and which of these are less relevant.

The exact weights of each objective are shown in the appendix. (Feng and Keller (2006), p. 82)

A well proven method of developing weights in the case of KI distribution is the swing weight method, which has been used also in this decision problem. When developing weights with the swing weight method, the decision maker needs to determine which of the stated objectives are of the worst and then of the best value. After realizing the objective giving the highest increase of the overall value, the decision maker will identify the objective with the highest weight. This process is repeated until all of the objectives get a certain weight. (Belton, Steward (2002), p. 135)

5.3.5. Value gaps

Value gaps give the decision maker the opportunity to see the differences between the current situation and the best possible set up and also to see the most significant areas of improvement easily. To demonstrate them we use the following table.

Table 3: Value gaps example

Objectives hierarchy	Weights (%)	No KI distribution	Value gaps	Ranking of value gaps
Minimize radiation health risks to public				
Minimize radioactive iodine risk to thyroid (51%)				
Maximize KI availability (26%)				
For children and pregnant women residents	20	0	2.0	1
For other residents	2	0	0.2	9
For mobile population	4	0	0.4	6
Optimize ability to take KI on time (16%)				
Number of people who know where KI is	5	0	0.5	3
Optimal time if no evacuation	5	0	0.5	3
Optimal time if evacuation	3	0	0.3	7
Storage to ensure stability	3	0	0.3	7
Minimize harm from inappropriate KI administration (9%)				
Correct dose given (and taken) for age	5	0	0.5	3
First dose not taken too late	3	10	0	11
Adverse side effects (nonthyroid cancer) minimized	1	10	0	11
Minimize harm from other aspects of the incident (49%)				
Minimize harm pre-incident (11%)				
Avoid excessive resources use in KI procedures	1	10	0	11
Educate public to respond to nuclear incident	10	0	1	2
Minimize harm during incident (38%)				
KI procedures do not impede evacuation	10	10	0	11
Avert mortality and morbidity from radiation or accidents	18	10	0	11
Minimize panic and anxiety due to KI procedures	2	5	0.1	10
Simplify KI procedures before and during incident	8	10	0	11

Source: Own representation with reference to Feng and Keller (2006), p. 83

14

No KI distribution is considered to represent the current situation. The best possible set up is a set up where all objectives are fully met, i.e. where each objective is reaching the rating of 10. Using the example objective „educate public to respond to nuclear incident", the value gaps can be calculated as follows:

$$w_i * (i - c) = g$$
$$10\% * (10 - 0) = 1$$

The term w_i represents the weight of the chosen objective and is multiplied with the difference of the ideal situation (i) with the current situation (c). The equation delivers the value gap (g) that can be used to improve the current situation. In the last column of the table 3 there is a ranking of the value gaps starting with the objective with the largest value gap, which is maximizing KI availability for children and pregnant women residents. It is very important for this analysis to understand that some of the objectives aren't delivering any value gaps. This is the case because some of them are fulfilled in the current situation. Fulfilled in the current situation are the objectives „first dose not taken too late", „adverse side effects (nonthyroid cancer) minimized", „avoid excessive resources use in KI procedures", „KI procedures do not impede evacuation", „avert mortality and morbidity from radiation or accidents" and „simplify KI procedures before and during incident". Furthermore as there are some trade-offs between the stated objectives, no alternative can fulfill all of them. The alternatives will be chosen according to the value gaps in the next step of this decision analysis. As already seen, it is possible that the current situation will perform better on some objectives than the chosen alternatives. (Feng and Keller (2006), p. 82-84)

5.3.6. Alternatives

Three alternatives have been chosen in this decision analysis in order to fulfill the stated objectives. They are shown in table 4.

Table 4: Alternative plan for the KI decision problem

Plans	Description
MM	Predistribute KI tablets inserted in mass mailing to households in KI planning zone (KIPZ), additional stockpiles at reception centers
VP	Predistribute to individuals in KIPZ via voluntary pickup, additional stockpiles at evacuation centers outside KIPZ
RC	Stockpile at evacuation reception centers outside KIPZ

Source: Own representation with reference to Feng and Keller (2006), p. 84

The first two alternatives mass mailing and voluntary pickup (MM and VP) have been chosen to reach the objectives with the highest value gaps. Both concentrate on maximizing the KI availability in the potential geographic region of a nuclear incident and also on optimizing the ability to take KI on time. The third alternative reception centers (RC) has been developed because the predistribution of KI tables also includes some disadvantages. The problem areas of the predistribution are mostly the specification of the predistribution area, correct instructions for taking and storing KI. The alternative RC, stockpiling KI at evacuation reception centers outside the KI planning zone, can help to make KI available to the affected population in the right area. This alternative also doesn't allow using excessive KI resources and helps to keep a track on the KI administration. (Feng and Keller (2006), p. 85)

5.3.7. Evaluation and decision

The last step of this decision analysis involves the alternative's evaluation together with presenting the recommendations. It begins with evaluating the objectives in all four alternatives. As mentioned above the alternative ND, no distribution, is also considered to be one of the alternatives and is thus also taken into account. The evaluation is using rating scales shown in figure 3. The alternative MM ensures that 85% of the population has an extra dose of KI at home, which leads to a fact, that MM scores with the highest possible rating in the objective to maximize KI availability to children and pregnant women. When one alternative is dominant on all stated objectives, it is clearly considered to be the best one.

Figure 3: Evaluating the alternatives

Objectives hierarchy	Calculated normalized weights (sum=%)	Sliders to determine raw swing weights (0-100)	Raw swing weights (maximum=100, minimum=0)	How well each plan meets each objective (Rate from 0 to 10 = best)			
				MM	VP	RC	ND
Minimize radiation health risks to public							
Minimize radioactive iodine risk to thyroid (51%)							
Maximize KI availability (26%)							
For children and pregnant women residents	◄ ►						
For other residents	◄ ►						
For mobile population	◄ ►						
Optimize ability to take KI on time (16%)							
Number of people who know where KI is	◄ ►						
Optimal time if no evacuation	◄ ►						
Optimal time if evacuation	◄ ►						
Storage to ensure stability	◄ ►						
Minimize harm from inappropriate KI administration (9%)							
Correct dose given (and taken) for age	◄ ►						
First dose not taken too late	◄ ►						
Adverse side effects (nonthyroid cancer) minimized	◄ ►						
Minimize harm from other aspects of the incident (49%)							
Minimize harm pre-incident (11%)							
Avoid excessive resources use in KI procedures	◄ ►						
Educate public to respond to nuclear incident	◄ ►						
Minimize harm during incident (38%)							
KI procedures do not impede evacuation	◄ ►						
Avert mortality and morbidity from radiation or accidents	◄ ►						
Minimize panic and anxiety due to KI procedures	◄ ►						
Simplify KI procedures before and during incident	◄ ►						
Overall value (Sum product of weights times ratings)							

Source: Own representation with reference to Feng and Keller (2006), p. 86

As already demonstrated there is some trade-off between the objectives. Furthermore it's obvious that in such a case there will be no dominant alternative but a need to evaluate all of them separately. In order to do so, the overall value of each alternative will be in the following counted by multiplying the weight of an objective with the result of the rating scale on each objective and summed into an overall value. This value helps the decision makers to see the appropriate alternative on the first sight. The results are illustrated in figure 4.

Figure 4: Evaluation of alternatives

Figure 4: Evaluation of alternatives

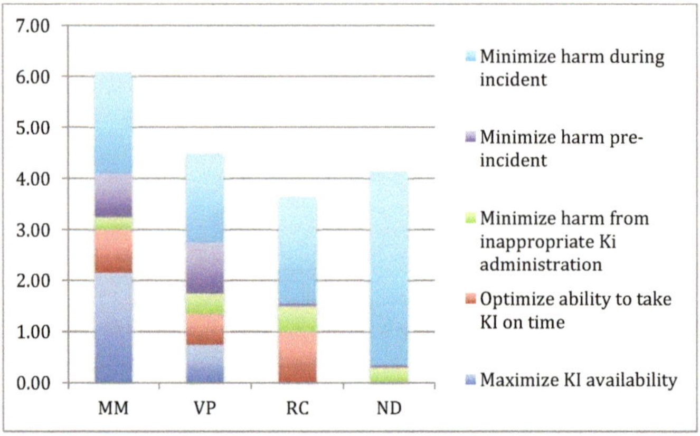

Source: Own representation with reference to Feng and Keller (2006), p. 86

All alternatives are divided into 5 subcategories that have been evaluated. The highest scoring achieves the alternative MM with 6,10 points followed by VP with 4,58, ND with 4,20 and RC with 3,77 points. As mentioned, MM, i.e. the KI predistribution scores with the most points and is therefore the recommended alternative. It helps to improve those objectives with the highest value gaps. Finally the decision maker can also think of new alternatives in order the improve those with the maximum reached points. (Feng and Keller (2006), p. 85-87)

6. Sensitivity Analysis

6.1. Sensitivity analysis in general

The term sensitivity analysis has different meaning in various communities and problem settings. „Until quite recently, sensitivity analysis was conceived and often defined as a local measure of the effect of a given input on a given output." (Saltelli et al. (2004), P. 42) This kind of analysis is often undertaken after conducting the decision tree analysis with the aim of proofing the reliability of the results. The main advantage of the sensitivity analysis is that it points out the demand for future research. It is of crucial importance to identify parameters that are uncertain and have impact on important decisions. These parameters can be then applied in further research. (Siebert (2003), p. 498, 500)

6.2. Tailor made analysis to specific contexts

This analysis is supposed to be executed in the hypothetical local region surrounded by the KI Planning Zone (KIPZ). The hypothetical local region could be every region in the vicinity of the plant, such as urban sites, suburban sites and rural areas. As these types of regions have different characteristics (i.e.: transportation, school and medical system, climate, etc.), there are also various decision problems in each of these regions as far as the distribution problem of KI is concerned. The same modeling framework for the decision analysis can be used in all regions mentioned, although the objectives hierarchy, alternatives, rating scales and so on may be different and influence the results of the KI distribution plan.

To sum up, it is essential to tailor made the analysis to the specific problem and context. In the multiple-objective decision analysis it is possible to use the same analysis process for generic types of problems and only adapt the objectives, alternatives and rating scales to the specific situation. (Feng and Keller (2006), p. 87-88)

6.3. One-Way Sensitivity Analysis

Generally speaking, the sensitivity analysis is a very appropriate tool in decisions with a single objective. The NRC committee prepared a one-way sensitivity analysis also for this potassium iodide multiple-objective decision analysis creating sliders in Microsoft Excel. The swing weight method (Figure 3) allows the researcher to perform a dynamic sensitivity analysis in decisions under certainty. This method allows the researcher to simply move the sliders of raw weights in Excel and ask „What if?" questions in order to analyze the problem in more detail and improve the decision making process. As far as the sensitivity analysis in multiple objective decisions is concerned, there are only few software options from which to choose.

Figure 3 presents a simple example with sliders that allow conducting sensitivity analysis with multiple objectives in the KI problem. Figure 3 consists of a sliders with the scale from 0 to 100 in order to determine raw swing weights (in the appendix please find attached the completed Excel spreadsheet). Changing the raw swing weight on one objective, does not automatically change the raw swing weights on other objectives. The change of raw weights will lead to variation in normalized weights. One of the advantages of the swing weight method is, that it makes possible to the stakeholders to look at bar graphs produced by Microsoft Excel and see, how variations in the weight of one objective changes the preferences among the different options. For example, changing the weight of the objective „Availability of KI" will automatically change the order of the most preferred distribution options MM, VP, RC, ND with the aim of meeting the objective.

The one-way sensitivity analysis for the KI problem will be demonstrated on two objectives from the decision analysis with the largest value gaps: „maximize KI availability for children and pregnant women residents" (abbreviation: „Availability") and „educate the public to respond to a nuclear incident" (abb.: „Education").

First of all, the one-way sensitivity analysis on the „Availability" objective will be performed for the purpose of finding out how the overall values of different distribution possibilities (MM, VP, RC, ND) vary when changing the raw swing weight on the „availability" objective. The raw weight for the „Availability" objective is set at 0, 50 and 100 and the normalized weight at 0 %, 11 % and 20 %. The raw weights are swinged while leaving other raw weights constant (at their base-case value). The raw as well as the normalized weights are shown in the appendix. Increasing the weight of the „Availability" objective, MM seems to perform the best. This is actually not surprising, as the predistribution of the potassium iodide in mass mailings will ensure and maximize the availability of KI for children and pregnant women in the affected area. Because of this fact, the MM option scores the best with the value of 10 compared to other alternative distribution possibilities of KI (VP value 2, RC value 2, ND value 0). In case, when the „Availability" objective has the raw weight of 0 (this objective has no importance), the ND option wins. Naturally speaking, if it is not crucial for the stakeholders to make KI available, the „No KI distribution" option will be chosen.

Figure 5: One-Way Sensitivity Analysis on Raw Swing Weight of „Availability" Objective

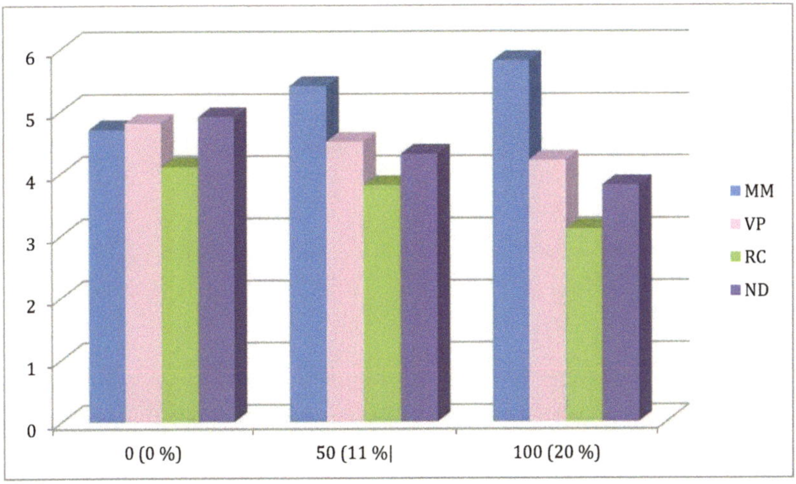

Source: Own representation with reference to Feng and Keller (2006), p. 89

Secondly, the one-way sensitivity analysis will be shown on the „Education" objective while varying the normalized weight from 0 to 1.0 (other than by „Availability" objective range 0 to 0,2) in order to get more deep insights into the problem. The main goal is to find out how the change of the normalized weight on the „Education" objective will influence the performance of the different distribution options of KI. All the other objectives will retain their base weights. If the normalized weight of the „Education" objective increases, the value for MM and VP option rises. On the other hand, by increase of the weight of the „Education" objective, the options RC and ND became less attractive. Furthermore, by raising the „Education" weight over 0,49, the VP option wins over all other alternatives with the rating value of 10. Again, there is a sense behind this result, as the people that pick up KI voluntary are more interested to be also educated about it. On the other hand, when the weight of the „Education" objective remains on the level 0,1, the MM option wins, like in the base-case scenario. (Figure 4) (Feng and Keller (2006), p. 88-90)

Figure 6: One-Way Sensitivity Analysis on Normalized Weight of „Education" Objective

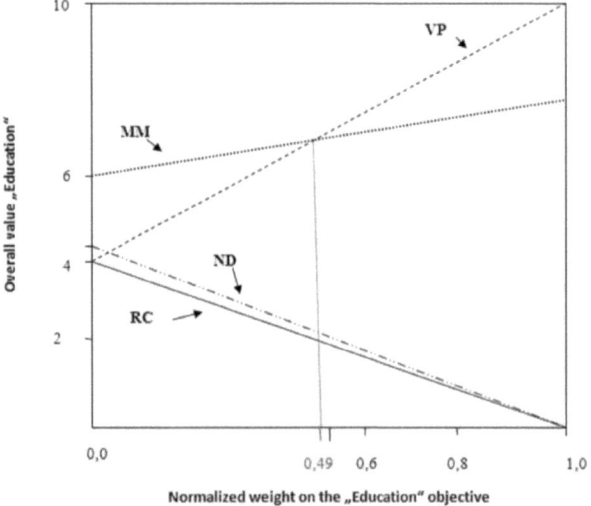

Source: Own representation with reference to Feng and Keller (2006), p. 89

6.4. Two-Way Sensitivity Analysis

The two-way sensitivity analysis in multiple-objective decisions is performed in a similar way as one-way sensitivity analysis. The only difference is that the weights of two (instead of one) objectives are varied and it is observed, how the performance of various alternatives changes.

Once again, the two objectives with the largest value gaps („Availability" and „Education") from the decision analysis will be used as a basis for administering the two-way sensitivity analysis. The raw swing weights of these two objectives will be swinged from 0 to 100, while leaving the raw weights of other objectives unchanged.

Figure 7: Two-Way Sensitivity Analysis on the „Availability" Objective and the „Education" Objective in the
KI Decision Problem

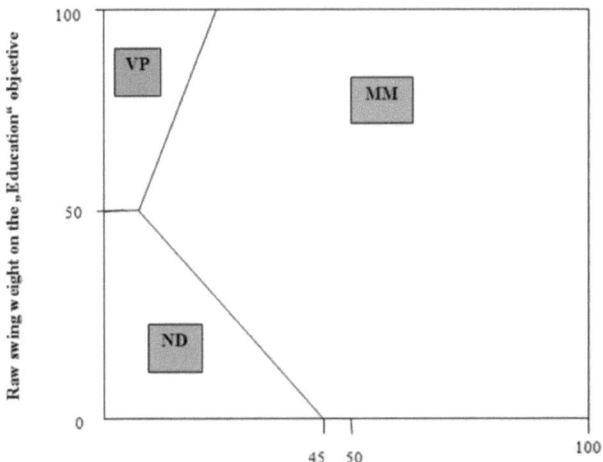

Raw swing weight on the „Availability" objective

Source: Own representation with reference to Feng and Keller (2006), P. 90

Figure 7 shows the two-way sensitivity analysis on the „Availability" and „Education" objectives for the hypothetical local region. By increasing the raw weight on the „Availability" objective the MM option (predistribution of KI in mass mailings) becomes the recommended choice no matter whether the weight of „Education" objective is high or low.

In case, the weight on the „Availability" as well as the „Education" objective is low, the status quo alternative (ND – no KI distribution) is preferred. Naturally speaking, if there is no interest among stakeholders in availability of KI and education about KI, no distribution of potassium iodide will be chosen.

On the other hand, the predistribution of KI via voluntary pickup (VP option) becomes preferable when the weight on the „Education" objective is high and the weight on the „Availability" objective is low (below 45). Voluntary pickup of KI would ensure a high quality of education, but many people would leave their doses unpicked thus reducing the „Availability" objective.

Figure 7 does not show the last option, the distribution of KI via stockpile at evacuation reception centers (RC option), because this alternative would be never recommended for the hypothetical local region in this base case.

To summarize, depending on the stakeholder objectives (low/high „Availability" or „Education") MM, ND and VP are the possible options for the hypothetical local region. (Feng and Keller (2006), p. 90)

7. Decision under uncertainty: A decision tree model

The NRC committee decided to focus on the decision analysis under certainty. Another possibility could be to analyze the problem using different techniques, i.e. decision trees. In order to be able to solve the decision-under-risk problem with decision trees, it would be necessary to assess the probabilities about key uncertainties and compute the costs of different KI distribution alternatives. A decision tree could be created with the aim of putting together sequences of uncertain events thus allowing calculating the probability of an entire path. This path would begin with a nuclear disaster and end with the release of radioiodine to the environment leading to certain financial and health consequences, which would be assessed in terms of health outcomes and monetary costs (i.e.: costs of the KI production and purchase, the number of affected population provided with KI, the number of KI doses to be available for one person, etc.). Averted thyroid cancer morbidity or mortality due to the administration of KI, averted or indirectly caused morbidity or mortality due to the nuclear accident or adverse health effects of KI medicine are the possible health outcomes, which would be included in the decision tree. (Feng and Keller (2006), p. 90-91)

The decision tree could look like as follows:

Figure 8: Decision tree for KI distribution

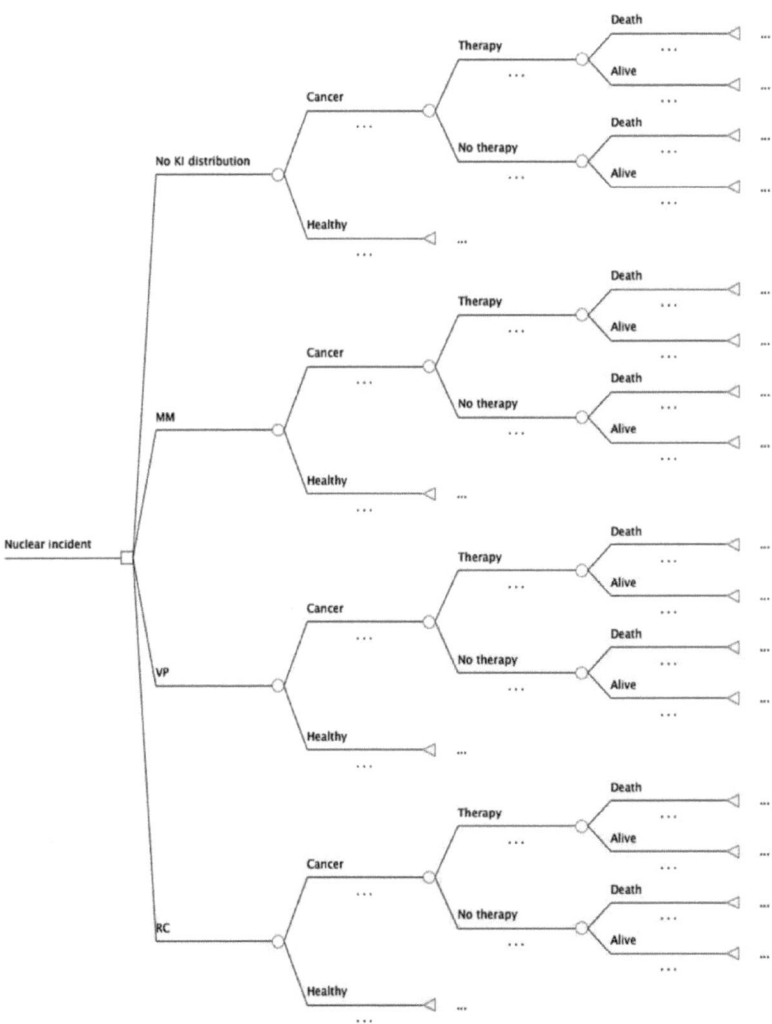

Source: Own representation

8. Similar studies

In general terrorism protection is of crucial importance for many countries, mainly after the attacks of September 11th. The potential threat of nuclear attacks is also increasing. As a result there exist a number of studies focusing on these matters.

The study "Assessment of Potassium Iodide (KI) Distribution Campaign and Emergency Response Around New Jersey's Nuclear Power Facilities" conducted by Blando et al. (2002) aims at evaluating the success of the KI distribution campaign in 2002 and the preparedness of the general public and emergency responders for nuclear disasters. The methodologies of this study were two written surveys, the first one designed for the general public and the second one for emergency responders. The results of the study unveiled that there is a lack of knowledge among both respondent groups regarding emergency preparedness for nuclear disasters. (Blando et al. 2002)

Another study dealing with the terrorism protection is the study "Balancing Terrorism and Natural Disasters – Defensive Strategy with Endogenous Attacker Effort" conducted by Zhuang and Bier. In this study the game theory was applied in order to come up with equilibrium strategies for attacker and defender in a case of terrorism and natural disasters. Furthermore it shows the protection balance from terrorism as well as natural disasters. In the center there is the description of the attacker's choice, which is measured by his level of effort. In the following the attacker can choose between increasing and decreasing his effort, which has an impact on the protection investments. (Zuang and Bier (2007), p. 976)

9. Conclusion

In summary, the use of the swing weight method for the multiple-objective decision analysis for terrorism protection allows the researcher to conduct a dynamic analysis and look at the problem from different perspectives. The extensive sensitivity analysis, which has been conducted by the NRC committee pointed out, that there is no single distribution plan suitable for all regions (urban sites, suburban sites, rural sites). As these areas are different from each other in a number of terms, the raw weights of objectives would be differently allocated thus leading to distinct solutions (recommended distribution paths of KI). For this reason, it is essential to conduct the multiple-objective decision analysis for each region separately.

The researcher committee presented in this paper a very interesting model for multiple-objective decisions under certainty. However, they rejected to compute costs of the various KI distribution methods and to assess the probabilities of key uncertainties for the purpose of conducting decision-under-risk analysis. Therefore it was not possible to carry out the cost-effectiveness analysis by constructing the CER Diagram or to fully take the advantage of the TreeAge Software for sensitivity analysis with the view of analyzing the specific KI problem with different methods and comparing the results.

Appendix: Sample Data to Evaluate Different Alternatives for a Hypothetical Local Region

Objectives	Normalized weights (Sum=100%) (%)	Raw Weights (100 =max, 0=min)	MM	VP	RC	ND
Minimize radiation health risks to public						
Minimize radioactive iodine risk to thyroid (51%)						
Maximize KI availability (26%)						
For children and pregnant women residents	20	100	10	2	0	0
For other residents	2	10	10	1	0	0
For mobile population	4	20	0	10	0	0
Optimize ability to take KI on time (14%)						
Number of people who know where KI is	5	25	0	5	10	0
Optimal time if no evacuation	3	25	10	3	0	0
Optimal time if evacuation	3	15	10	10	10	0
Storage to ensure stability	3	15	0	0	10	0
Minimize harm from inappropriate KI administration (9%)						
Correct dose given (and taken) for age	5	25	0	5	10	0
First dose not taken too late	3	15	10	10	0	10
Adverse side effects (nonthyroid cancer) minimized	1	5	0	8	10	10
Minimize harm from other aspects of incident (49%)						
Minimize harm pre-incident (11%)						
Avoid excessive resources use in KI procedures	1	5	0	5	7	10
Educate public to respond to nuclear incident	10	50	8	10	0	0
Minimize harm during incident (38%)						
KI procedures do not impede evacuation	10	50	0	5	10	10
Avert mortality and morbidity from radiation or accidents	18	90	10	3	0	10
Minimize panic and anxiety due to KI procedures	2	10	10	5	10	5
Simplify KI procedures before and during incident	8	40	0	3	10	10
Sum of weights	100	500				
Overall value **(sum product of weights times ratings)**			6,10	4,58	3,77	4,20

Source: Own representation with reference to Feng and Keller (2006), P. 92

List of book references

Belton, B.; Steward, T. J. „*Multiple Criteria Decision Analysis, An Integrated Approach.*"
1. Auflage, Kluwer Academic Publishers 2002.

Bennett, B.; Repacholi, M.; Carr, Z. „*Health Effects of the Chernobyl Accident and Special Health Care Programmes.*" WHO – World Health Organization. Report of the UN Chernobyl Forum, Expert Group "Health". Geneva 2006.

Feng, T.; Keller, L. R. „*A Multiple-Objective Decision Analysis for Terrorism Protection: Potassium Iodide Distribution in Nuclear Incidents.*" Decision Analysis. Informs 2006, Vol. 3, No. 2, pp. 76-93.

Feng, T. et al. „*Modeling Multi-Objective Multi-Stakeholder Decisions: A Case-Exercise Approach*" Informs 2008, Vol. 8, No. 3, pp. 103-114.

National Research Council of the National Academies. „*Distribution and administration of potassium iodide in the event of a nuclear incident.*" 1. Auflage, Washington, The National Academies Press 2004.

Saltelli, A.; Tarantola, S.; Campologno, F.; Ratto, M. „*Sensitivity analysis in practice. A guide to assessing scientific models.*" 1. Auflage, Chichester, John Wiley & Sons, Ltd 2004.

Schwartz, F. W. et al. „*Das Public Health Buch, Gesundheit und Gesundheitswesen.*" 2. Auflage, Urban & Fischer, München-Jena 2003.

Siebert, U. „*Transparente Entscheidungen in Public Health mittels systematischer Entscheidungsanalyse.*" Urban & Fischer, München 2003.

Zhuang, J.; Bier, V. M. „*Balancing Terrorism and Natural Disasters - Defensive Strategy with Endogenous Attacker Effort.*" Operations Research. Informs 2007, Vol. 55, No. 5, pp. 976–991.

List of internet references

Blando, J. et al. „*Assessment of Potassium Iodide (KI) Distribution Campaign and Emergency Response Around New Jersey's Nuclear Power Facilities.*" 2002. http://www.nj.gov/health/surv/documents/ki_finalrpt.pdf (Access on September 19th 2012).

REMM – Radiation Emergency Medical Management, U.S. Department of Health and Human Services. „*Potassium Iodide (KI).*" December 2011. http://www.remm.nlm.gov/potassiumiodide.htm (Access on August 24th 2012).

WNA - World Nuclear Association. „*Chernobyl Accident 1986.*" April 2012. http://www.world-nuclear.org/info/chernobyl/inf07.html (Access on August 14th 2012).

WNA – World Nuclear Association. „*Fukushima Accident 2011.*" August 2012. http://www.world-nuclear.org/info/fukushima_accident_inf129.html (Access on August 26th).

YOUR KNOWLEDGE HAS VALUE

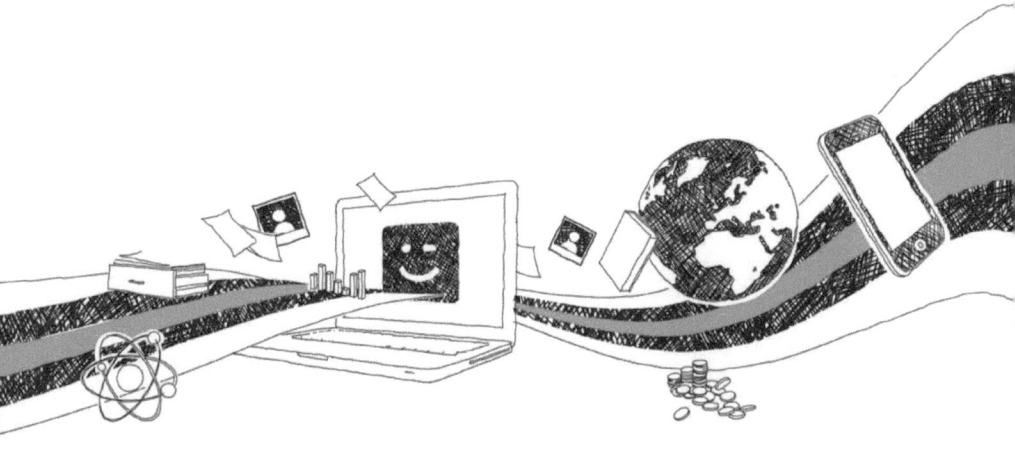

- We will publish your bachelor's and
  master's thesis, essays and papers

- Your own eBook and book -
  sold worldwide in all relevant shops

- Earn money with each sale

Upload your text at www.GRIN.com
and publish for free

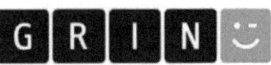